Hip Replacement Adaptive Equipment

and the Sport of Recovery
A Patient's Perspective

By Martin E. Dodge

Spring, thank you!!!

I am grateful for the support my wife Spring provides. She is my nurse during my recovery process. Spring is my first reader and viewer of the content I create. I learn the skills to make this book, videos, website, and other subjects related to this endeavor as I go. The learning curve is steep, and Spring cautions me to take breaks, so I will not burn out and lose sight of why I am doing this project. She always sets me back on the path of creating the best quality content I can produce.

Table of Contents

Book Key, Disclaimers, Credits, and Copyright Information

Key for reading this book

- ➢ Orthopaedics vs. Orthopedics: both words are correct. My doctor prefers "Orthopaedics."
- ➢ Adaptive Equipment items are <u>C</u>apitalized throughout the book.
- ➢ Bordered text boxes provide additional narration and storytelling.
- ➢ Watch my videos on YouTube (see how in References.)
- ➢ The author does not claim any rights to the operating room video, "Minimally invasive anterior hip arthroplasty, the Röttinger approach - Dr. O. Bringer." The video has a YouTube Creative Commons Attribution license (reuse allowed). A YouTube address for the operating room video is listed in the References section.

Medical Disclaimer

The author of this book is not a medical professional and is sharing a personal experience. The reader should pursue accredited professional medical assistance regularly and follow all treatment guidelines provided by a licensed medical doctor.

Credits

Book design and production by Martin E. Dodge
Editing by Leni Williams
Photography and video by Martin E. Dodge

Foreword

The goal of this book is to create the guidebook I could not find to soothe my nerves, educate, and prepare me for hip replacement surgery. My medical program does not provide outcome scenarios ahead of the surgery; it promotes a shopping list and a checklist of appointments leading up to the big day. Patients are expected to plan ahead for mobility challenges at home and acquire the recommended Adaptive Equipment to use during the recovery process. I shine a light on the list of Adaptive Equipment I use and review similar items with hands on experience. I hope my story helps prospective patients plan for their comfort and adjustment to life after hip replacement surgery.

There are many books and sources of information where authors detail their expertise, and personal experience to write an account of hip replacement surgery. Some authors have had the operation themselves but fall into the trappings of medical validation by focusing on operating room information and listing the stuff you will be prompted to buy but skip the recovery process. Humor and personal stories add a humanizing note, but the levity does not reassure me as a prospective patient.

If you need to have hip replacement surgery, I am guessing you do not want to remember what takes place in the operating room and you are more concerned with what life is like after. I provide a patient perspective of my recovery comparing the Adaptive Equipment I use during my healing process. Your experience will be unique, but we share a common recovery process and a list of stuff to use.

YouTube is a resource I use to find information in addition to reading. Surprisingly, videos produced by hospital programs tend to be awkward. Interns do not make good patient models. The disorienting atmosphere caused by opioids, sleep deprivation, and mobility challenges cannot be role-played by not-patients, and the setting of the videos never represent a home environment where rehabilitation actually occurs.

I thank all of the patients who made videos for sharing their stories. Videos created by actual patients are on point with movement details, but they tend to be wordy. I am guilty of that tendency considering I decided to write this book, oops. I present my own videos to provide precise instructions concerning the activities I highlight using text captions.

The patient's financial concerns are overlooked by the medical community, and I do not have a solution to offer. I opt to pay for the surgery with a monthly payment plan the hospital offers that is zero interest added to the amount owed. I have insurance, and for me, the surgery equals buying a "good" used car that happens to be my body. The reader must seek out the best way to make the surgery happen unless life in a wheelchair is an acceptable resolution.

I need to change my occupation to better accommodate my body after the surgery. I was not informed of the possibility I would need to change my career, and there is a lot to figure out how to make that a reality. Despite the surprise employment realization, I do not regret enjoying the benefits hip replacement surgery has given me.

Hip Replacement Adaptive Equipment

and the Sport of Recovery

A Patient's Perspective

By Martin E. Dodge

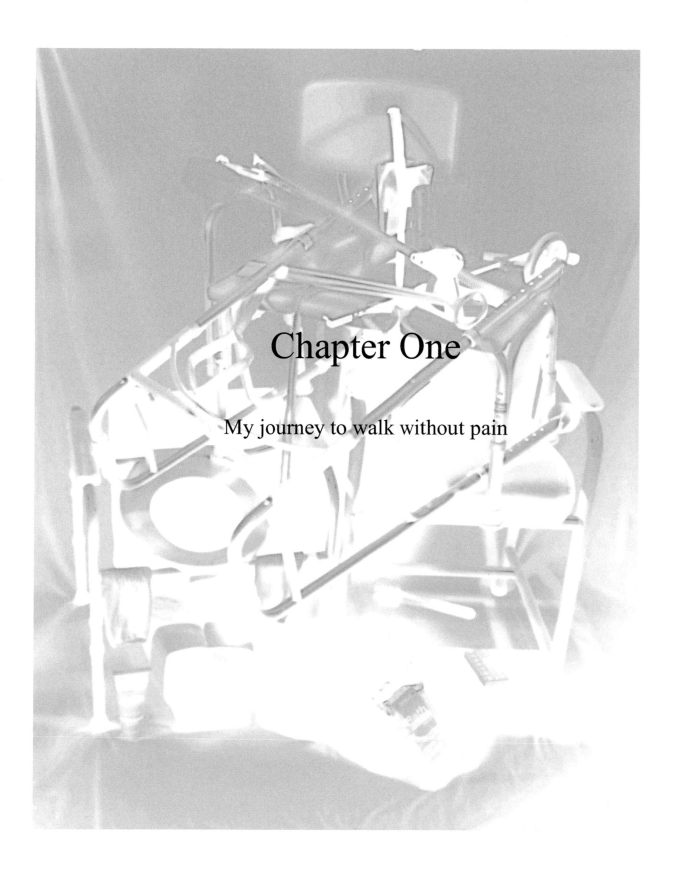

Chapter One

My journey to walk without pain

My journey to walk without pain

I do not realize the extent or nature of my hip problem for years. The initial injury happens in 2009, a very stressful year for me, and I cause it while sleeping. I awake in a specific range of body contortion positions several times. The aspects of the contortions are that my right leg is bent crooked at a sharp angle, my body while asleep then turns to add mounting pressure to the leg where it meets the hip socket. This body position cuts off the blood flow to my right hip joint and at the same time forces some separation of my leg from the socket. I wake up in pain lying face down with my arms tucked under me, and they are uselessly asleep. I rock my body side to side until my arms are free and wait for blood flow to restore feeling and the ability to use my arms to straighten my right leg and then wait for the leg to pop itself back into place. I awake in this situation several times. A bone deteriorating disease, osteonecrosis, develops in my right hip's skeletal ball joint as a result of this unconscious posturing; it is an irreversible process and the only solution to avoid being wheelchair dependent is a hip replacement surgery. I begin my journey to walk without pain in 2016.

The stressful time gradually diminishes, and I do not awake in extreme positions. Life goes on as usual, but the leg becomes painful in various ways over time. I think the problem is with my knee because it is the loudest voice of complaint from the problem leg most of the time. Using a compression wrap alleviates the pain from the knee area until I start working a job that has me standing in place for long periods. I stand with my weight oriented on the leg that doesn't bother me to reduce pressure and pain as a solution. Chiropractic therapy is my first choice when my hip and leg really start to be an issue, and its treatment helps a significant number of things. The chiropractor tells me to get an X-ray when efforts to relieve pain in the hip area no longer provide relief.

I go to a general practitioner doctor for a physical and to express my concerns about my hip and leg. The doctor sends me to get an X-ray of my hips before I leave and refers me to the orthopaedic department after reviewing the image. The official diagnosis takes place after another X-ray is requested and viewed by an orthopaedic surgeon's assistant. I am already aware of the worst possible diagnosis, but I am unprepared for the news that both hips need to be replaced. The problem hip is in a horrible condition, and the other hip is in an early stage of the same degenerative process. I decide to do one hip at a time and plan a timeline for surgery.

The advancing intensity of pain inspires me to learn new ways of moving and walking to minimize my discomfort while I work. I need to save money to get me through the time away from work I need to recover from surgery. Mobility becomes more a study of how not to move. Standing for lengths of time is very painful, and I work on my feet. I am scheduled to work full time, but I can only handle part-time hours. The pain is too big a nuisance to disguise, so I set the time for my surgery at the start of the slow season at work. I have three months to prepare.

The medical program provides a class to inform patients on what to expect. A nurse coordinator shows a presentation of what the surgical procedure is in graphic detail and deflects answers to many post-surgery concerns, including the use of the Adaptive Equipment featured, to instruction from an occupational therapist who will consult with patients after their procedure. I leave the class with a Patient Program Guidebook that contains details of how to prepare, Adaptive Equipment to get, exercise to do before and after, what to do in general, and lists to help patients organize. The class provides patients with a swag bag containing lip balm, special soap, and body-wipes to be used starting three days before the surgery.

I borrow a walker from family and visit a range of places to compare prices and variety for the other Adaptive Equipment the class mentions and pictures in the Patient Program Guidebook. All the items on the list are of a short-term need of nature. There is no guarantee Goodwill, or the Salvation Army will have anything, but it is worth a look to economize collecting the list of items. A local medical supply store and Walmart are options, but Amazon.com ultimately wins me over with easy browsing and suggested items. The design and practicality of some items do not qualify, in my opinion, to be necessary purchases. I will provide details concerning the Adaptive Equipment later in this book.

Some legal paperwork needs to be completed before the surgery can take place. The medical program provides me with an Advanced Directive Form that I must register before any procedure. This is my first such form, so I need to get signatures from my family members or a person I select to represent me to authenticate the form. This is an opportunity to make sure information is up to date if I already have such a document and remind any person of their potential role in the form. I make copies of the signed form to give them to all persons involved. The medical program provides directions concerning what forms and information I will need to bring with me for any procedures.

Just to be safe in the unlikely event my surgery goes horribly wrong, I go to the bank with my wife to sign a form stating she has control of my checking and savings accounts should I pass away. We maintain separate accounts, and without this step, my wife would find it difficult to recover the assets I would like to leave her. I would do this even if we had joint accounts just in case something needs both of our signatures. I also provide my wife with a list of all my online accounts that involve bank account access or credit card use with usernames, passwords, security questions, and answers.

A week before surgery, I see an anesthesiologist who informs me of my options and makes suggestions to maximize my comfort (or dare I say blissful ignorance of what is happening to me) in the operating room. I am required to bring a copy of the Advanced Directive Form and sign more forms stating my agreement to the services the anesthesiologist will provide in the operating room.

Leading up to the final month before surgery, I stop taking vitamins, supplements, and Advil in stages. I also begin taking a mild stool softener, a week before surgery, to prepare for constipation caused by Oxycodone, and baby Aspirin as a blood thinner to reduce the chance of fatal blood clots. A bathing routine with anti-bacterial/microbial soap is the last step in the process leading to the big event. I make sure to review the materials provided by the medical program and check off a list of things to do and have done before I need to leave for the hospital. My hospital stay bag is ready to travel the night before surgery.

The night before I must not eat after 11:00 p.m. and drink only small amounts of water beyond that time, but I can consume a 16-ounce bottle of Gatorade on the way to the hospital before surgery; I am told this will ease some discomfort later in the day. Before leaving to go to the hospital the day of surgery, I do a final scrub with the special soap and body wipes.

Checking into the hospital reminds me of an airport, though boarding is where the similarity ends. The waiting room has a check-in desk where you are assigned a number to be notified when you can proceed to the next area for surgery preparation. There are lockers available to stow items I can have family or other representatives retrieve later. Televisions displaying patient's names and procedure progress are placed around the large room filled with hopeful bodies and souls waiting for progress. My wait is mercifully short.

I am led to a preparation room where I surrender my earthly possessions, don a surgical gown, and hairnet, and get outfitted with IV attachments to feed my body drugs and fluids for the stages of procedures that come next. Before I am wheeled out of the preparation room, I sign paperwork confirming what is to be done and a member of the surgical team stops in to sign on my body with a marker where the team will begin work.

My clothing and any forms or information I bring into this room do not go with me to the operating room. My wife collects my belongings and goes to the family waiting room, a separate space from the check-in room, while I am in surgery. A television in the room displays updates for family and care providers on a list of patients undergoing procedures during and concluding operations.

The YouTube address for the surgery video is listed in the References section of this book if you need it.

My wife is at my bedside in a holding area when I wake up in the afternoon. I am given a cocktail of drugs to ease my pain, which fuels my sense of time distortion and other cognitive abnormalities. The boredom and discomfort of my wife have no offer of being remedied, though. She is a saint; I am blessed to have her. She reminds me later the doctors attending the holding area did provide me with some ginger ale, which I shared with her.

A long wait for a bed to be moved to from the holding area ensues. When I am moved to a bed, food service is no longer available. I have not eaten from 10:45 p.m. the night before the surgery until after 5:30 p.m. following the surgery because of the wait for a bed to become available. A physical therapist notices I am very shaky while coaching me how to get in and out of bed. I state the cause as low blood sugar, and the need for me to eat as the cure, to stop whatever plan to save me is initiated.

Bringing a bag of candy for your hospital stay is not a hunger or blood sugar solution. Luckily, my wife is with me to insist I need to eat. Please, have someone who can advocate for your condition and get you nourishment. My wife goes out to get a sandwich for me, and after I eat it, I stop shaking. The hospital provides a good experience after my need to eat is established.

I am shown the features of the hospital bed to control the room lights, how to call for a nurse and operate the TV. My feet are fitted with motorized slippers that massage my soles to enhance blood circulation and reduce the risk of blood clots. A nurse shows me how to use an Incentive Spirometer to exercise my lungs to help recover from any effects of the anesthesia used during surgery. The over-night stay care schedule board posted on a wall in the room is explained to me before the physical therapist and attending nurse both leave. My wife bids me good night and returns to our home. I prepare to binge watch some Netflix on my tablet.

The drugs certainly help with surgical pain, but the familiar pain was no longer there. The need to drink plenty of fluids is reinforced with an intravenous drip that gets replenished a few times. Moving on and off the bed to pee was done often with minimal discomfort. For safety, any movement off of the bed was supervised by a nurse that I notified about the need with the push of a button. The nurse made sure I was safely back on the bed, too. Every four hours, a nurse brings the prescribed medications and makes sure I take them. The nurse always asks me about the level of pain I am experiencing and assists with the dosage to manage it. Halfway through the night, the nerve block injection I received shortly before surgery begins to wear off. The mounting pain caps off as no worse than what I was used to before surgery – but it is now constant and not randomly fluctuating. I accept the maximum dosage of Oxycodone from the nurse at the next medication time and am fine.

In the morning, after breakfast, a physical therapist guides me outside of the room to practice walking up and down stairs, getting into and out of a mock car, and monitors how my leg posture is while using a walker. I am told to be mindful of keeping the foot of the operative leg from turning inward. The process of training my muscles and other soft tissue to heal and rehabilitate correctly has begun. I pass the necessary mobility tests easily, and I am told an occupational therapist will visit with me in a little while to observe a few more mobility basics.

The occupational therapist brings some Adaptive Equipment items which I can take home if I do not already have them. This situation annoys me because I did ask if some items would be provided to patients during the preparation class I attended, and the response was a solid, "maybe." I prove the ability to use: A Leg Lifter Strap to get in and out of bed, a Sock Aid to put on socks, a Reacher Grabber Stick to put on pants, and a Long-Handled Shoehorn to put on shoes and take off socks. The therapist also makes sure I can use the commode with side handles in the bathroom adjacent to my bed within the room I have been assigned. I decide to keep some of the items: The Long-Handled Sponge – I didn't have one, and the Leg Lifter Strap, Sock Aid, and Reacher Grabber Stick – all different and more user-friendly than the items I had bought. The occupational therapist approves my readiness for release.

> The first two weeks of recovery are the hardest. The challenge of doing things lessens as new mobility behaviors become more familiar. With luck, the most inconvenient adjustment for you will be taking medication every four hours of every 24 hours. The quality of movement improves every week that passes, sometimes daily, and there is less to complain about. In perspective of how much complaining may have taken place before the surgery, the gains might be even greater.

The hospital provides the prescription fill for Oxycodone, up to a two-week prescription of 5-milligram tablets. Oxycodone is the painkiller for the recovery time after surgery, and I take it every four hours at a maximum of two pills. I get a two-week supply. The minimum dosage of this opioid-based medication is effective for managing my pain. I take the maximum dosage shortly before doing any exercise and maybe the next dosage time after exercising depending on how I feel. Extra Strength Tylenol is sufficient enough to manage my discomfort for the weeks that follow after the Oxycodone runs out.

I did not experience any swelling for a couple of days after surgery, which is unusual. Swelling in the operative leg is inevitable, though. The exercises and movements prescribed by the medical program must be done regularly to reduce swelling in addition to preventing the formation of blood clots. Doing the stretches and lying on my back with the operative leg raised is crucial to drain the fluid that collects in the lower portion of the operative leg. The frequency of this exercise is at least every half an hour to hour at first. I apply a large reusable ice pack to the surgery site for ten minutes after exercising.

Within two weeks, I attend a gym that specializes in outpatient physical therapy. The gym is a physical therapy provider approved by my medical program. The range of exercises increases in difficulty as I gain motor skill and strength. The physical therapy doctor provides me with additional exercises that I do at home in between my two visits a week. None of the exercises look hard to perform, but despite being simple tasks, they do require willpower to complete.

Six weeks after the surgery, I meet with the surgeon for the first follow up visit. I still have minor discomfort if I bend where I shouldn't. The surgeon says I should not lift more than forty pounds for the next three months. I can stop taking the last prescribed medication for surgery recovery, baby aspirin used as a blood thinner, and I have written permission to drive again. Daily physical therapy is an ongoing activity, but the need to go to a physical therapy gym will end soon, and progress in physical wellbeing will be up to my unsupervised choices.

I return to work three months after the surgery. During month four of my recovery, I pull a heavy object like I was normal, and it did not budge. Within an hour, I know I made a mistake and wonder if the ring of pain in my operative leg will subside with a little rest. I lose three days of work before I can get a checkup with my orthopaedic doctor. An X-ray reveals no damage to the bone. The pain is caused by internal swelling due to the fragile nature of tissues surrounding the implant around the bone at the surgery site. I am sent to get an ultrasound scan to search for blood clots in the operative leg as a safety precaution before I am cleared to return to work. The pain soon recedes, and I am extra careful not to repeat the experience.

Another checkup six months later provides me with a greater understanding of how use and stress will affect the new hip joint. I thought that as the bone strengthened its connection to the metal implant, there would be a return to a state of movement as before with some limitations. I was wrongly optimistic about the temporary nature of the forty-pound lifting limit. The construction of the implant contains a plastic cup that buffers impact the same way cartilage in the joint socket would if I still had it. The metal ball joint mashing into this plastic cup will cause damage to it and create the need for surgery to replace the part if care is not observed.

My post-surgery body is new to me, and I begin a process of learning and adjustment. I am a moderately active person, and the limitations of my new body thankfully don't affect walking or most of the kind of hiking I like to do. My kayaks weigh 60 pounds each, though, and I transport them on top of my car. This is an activity I refuse to give up so I will look into alternative ways to load them. I decide to pursue a job that is more friendly to the preservation of my hip implant. Work friends at my current job do tasks I am not able to perform when I ask them to, and I find ways to compensate for their help. The path ahead is challenging, but the ability to walk without pain is something to celebrate.

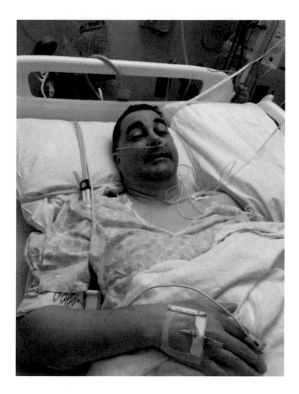

I am smiling, really! I am drugged up and freshly awake after surgery. My wife takes a picture with her phone to send to my family as proof that I am alive.

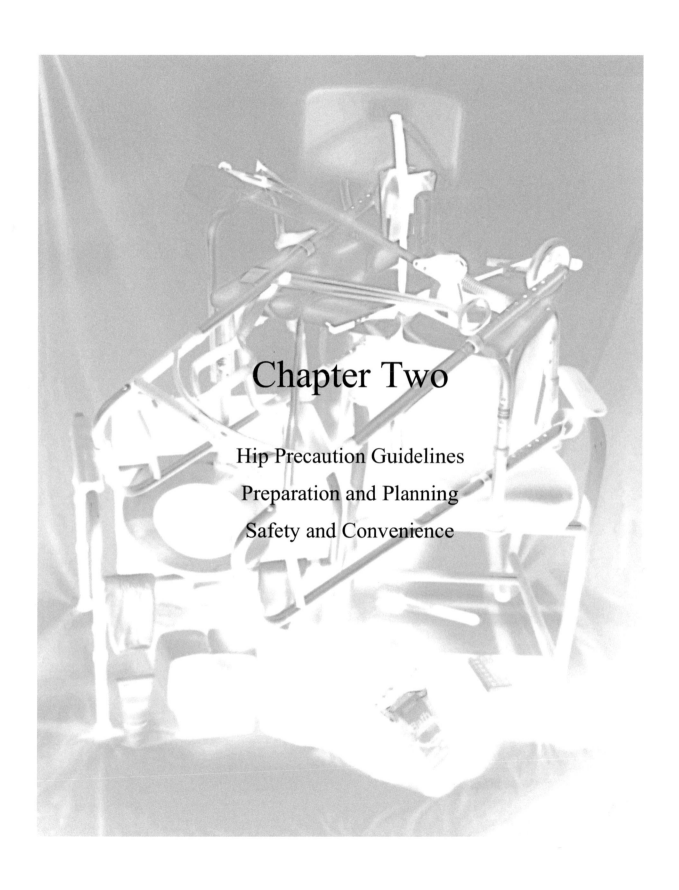

Chapter Two

Hip Precaution Guidelines

Preparation and Planning

Safety and Convenience

The following list is the standard set of instructions you will need to be mindful of after the surgery until you are fully recuperated.

Hip Precaution Guidelines

Do Not cross your legs

Do Not bend or lean forward

Do Not bend your hip past 90 degrees

Do Not turn your knee inward

Do:

Use your walker as advised by your doctor

Use your Raised Toilet Seat

Use pain/ discomfort as your guide in moving your surgery affected hip

Take walks using aids for added support and stability as needed

Preparation and Planning:

Prepare for before and after Surgery

The medical program for hip replacement surgery will provide many assurances and answers about what Adaptive Equipment to get and what to expect before and after surgery. You should attend any classes offered by the program and consult with your nurse coordinator if you have questions or concerns. Your priority is the most successful outcome possible for the surgery, and anything you can do to ensure it should be pursued. Learn about diet, exercise, self-control, and any source of information that will assist you in preparing for the procedure and adapting to your life after it.

Mental and Physical Preparation

The first and most crucial piece of Adaptive Equipment is you, the patient. You need to take control of your habits to ensure your best possible future. In short, quit doing anything bad for your health well before the surgery and be able to maintain that state until at least after you recover. If you feel you can't do this by yourself, please get help. Do not deceive yourself or your doctor about any addictions. Pursue a weight loss program if needed. I encourage you to take control of your life to restore your ability to walk without pain.

Prepare Yourself for Surgery Recovery Time

Several days before surgery, take care of needs that require going somewhere, such as hair, nails, or other grooming you can't do at home. Get styled in a way that does not need to be redone for six weeks. You will probably be able to get out of the house after a couple of weeks, but not on your own, and there is no guarantee a seat with Hip Precaution Guidelines will be waiting for you in public.

Boredom and cabin fever will be your constant companions unless you plan for activities and hobbies in addition to reading and binge watching. I formed the idea to outline this book as one of many things to do during my recovery time. I could not easily shake off cabin fever, though. Walking around the neighborhood gets you outside but not far enough away to feel like a break from being stuck at home. Try to have friends or family take you places to do more than get groceries when possible.

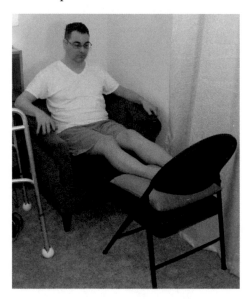

Safety and Convenience:

Prepare Home or Care Place for after the Surgery

○ Plan to leave the lights on or get night lights so you will always be able to see when moving around in the living space you will inhabit during your recovery from surgery.

○ Get the Adaptive Equipment items that you need and practice using and placing them in your recovery environment.

○ Secure any power cords, remove bathmats, loose rugs, and any other floor hazards that will be in the way of using a Walker.

○ Move items you frequently use to where you can effortlessly reach them, such as items stored high and low in cabinets, dresser drawers, closets, under sinks, and so on.

○ Food preparation should be made to be as easy as possible. Cook meals in advance to freeze and reheat, buy prepackaged meals or soups, and healthy snacks. Arrange help from family, friends, and coworkers to bring meals.

○ Plan for how and where you will eat. It is difficult to carry food and beverages while using a Walker. Standing at a counter to eat may be the best solution until you can walk with confidence.

○ Select the bed you will use ahead of the surgery. Measure the height of the bed from the floor to the top of the mattress, note the side of the bed you will use in relation to the operative leg, and make a record of this information to share with an occupational therapist. Plan to place items you will use frequently close to the bed, preferably within an arm's reach.

○ Set up the bathroom you plan to use with the necessary Adaptive Equipment. Make sure you can get in and out of the bathroom using a Walker. Determine if you need to install handles on a wall or in the shower for extra safety. Do not plan to use towel rods or other bath fixtures to support your weight.

○ The Raised Toilet Seat is the most essential item in the bathroom. Make sure the style of seat is appropriate and is correctly placed and adjusted for your comfort and safety.

○ If you have any questions or concerns about your physical needs and using Adapting Equipment at home, contact your nurse coordinator, or an appropriate professional about the issue before it is a problem.

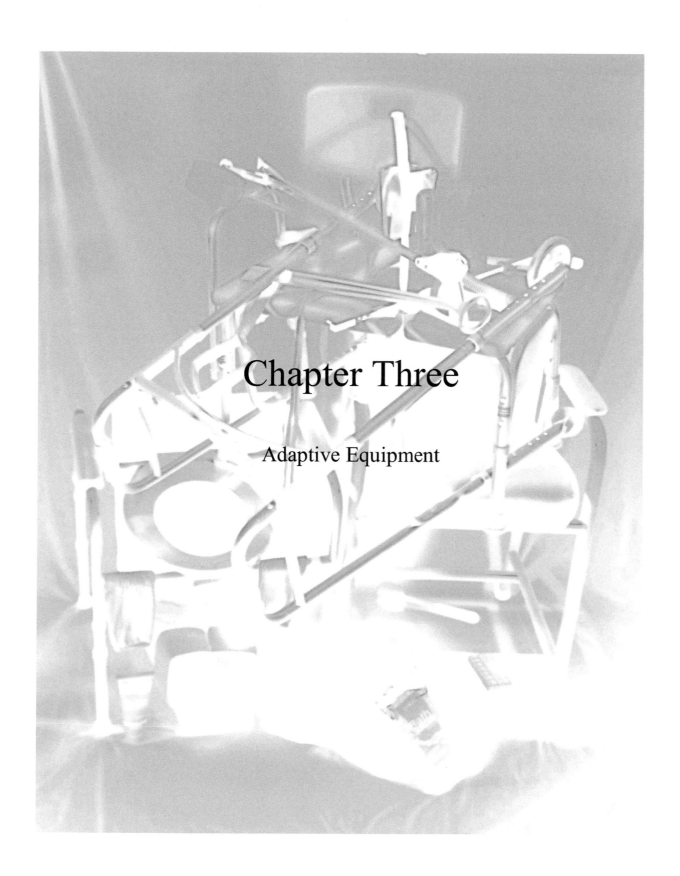

Chapter Three

Adaptive Equipment

Adaptive Equipment:

  The Adaptive Equipment my Patient Program Guide presents, and additional items that make my recovery from surgery more comfortable are in the following list. The items are separated into sections based on when they are needed during your journey. You can use this list as a checklist for shopping or form questions to ask your medical program about personal needs and concerns. I review similar items with commentary I glean from using the items. More information about using the Adaptive Equipment is included later on.

Items to bring with you to the hospital

○ Bag of candy

○ Chapstick – your lips will be irritated and very chapped after surgery (due to use of an oxygen tube)

○ Slippers with backs – not flip-flop style

○ Walking Shoes with Elastic Shoelaces

○ Pajamas, nightgown, short robe, underwear, socks, loose shorts, jogging suit, sweatpants, tops, etc.

○ Toothbrush, toothpaste, and any other toiletry comforts you usually use

>   I am discharged from the hospital the day after surgery, so I barely use any of the items I bring. During my stay in the hospital, I wear a hospital gown and stay on the bed, unless I need to call for help to get up and pee. I think I would use more items if I need to stay a second night. There is no way of knowing when you will be eligible for discharge, so just be prepared. I leave the hospital wearing the clothes I arrived in.

Elastic Shoelaces

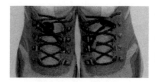

You will want to make putting your shoes on as easy as possible. Elastic shoelaces can be cut to fit your shoes and adjusted for comfort and hold.

Item to have brought for you on discharge day

Walker

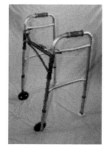

You will be delivered to your ride home in a wheelchair driven by orderlies, and they will assist you to get in the vehicle if you need. The Walker will ultimately get you back indoors from the car and be your best friend for a week.

Items you will bring home from the hospital

Incentive Spirometer

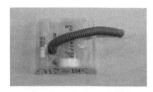

This item is used to exercise your lungs to help recover from any effects anesthesia used during surgery may cause. You inhale air through a tube intending to raise a floating level and maintain its position in a specific range. The exercise is repeated every 10 -15 minutes. This activity is a very brief part of recovery.

Foam Wedge

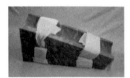

You will wake up with your legs strapped to a dense foam wedge. The wedge is used to keep your legs in an easier position to move you after surgery. I decided to keep the wedge to use so I wouldn't easily roll onto my side while sleeping. The wedge is also great for elevating the operative leg to reduce swelling.

Non-skid Socks

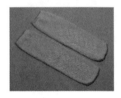

You will wake up from surgery wearing a hospital gown and a pair of non-skid socks. The socks provide traction for safety while walking in the hospital.

Items that may be offered to you at the hospital (have at home, do not plan on them being provided)

○ Long-handled Shoehorn

○ Reacher Grabber Stick

○ Leg Lifter

○ Sock Aid

○ Long-handled Sponge

Items to have waiting at home or care place

Have these items ready for you to use when you get home. Practice using the items before your surgery to make sure placement is as correct as possible.

Raised Toilet Seat – two styles are in the Adaptive Equipment list provided by the orthopaedic department

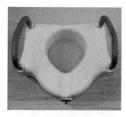 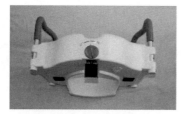

The orthopaedic department of which I am a patient offers no clear advice on which seat to buy.

Do not buy the seat that attaches to the commode. I found it inappropriate for my hip surgery recovery.

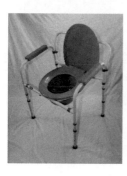 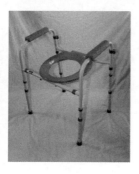

The other sits on top of its own frame, allowing it to be used away from the bathroom, and both styles of Raised Toilet Seats have handles to assist with sitting and getting up.

Buy the freestanding Raised Toilet Seat and adjust it for your comfort for use before you go to the hospital. The frame of the seat will fit around the commode without removing the existing seat and lid. I provide some personal experience as to why this is my seat of choice later.

In summary: you will pee with high frequency after the surgery, so if you need to sit down to do so be prepared. Your body will have difficulty producing bowel movements for a few days after surgery due to the opioid-based pain reducing medication Oxycodone, so when you need to go there should be no distraction from using this seat to achieve relief.

Reacher Grabber Stick
I have two kinds.

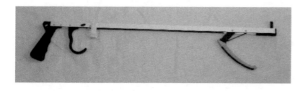

One for light use, it has a peg sticking out on its backside at the claw end that is useful for grabbing pants, socks, and other items when the grabber claw is too big. This is my preferred Reacher Grabber.

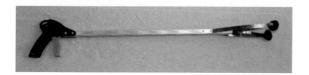

One for heavier lifting, it is mostly made of metal parts and has suction cups on the tips of the grabber claw. I feel this style of Reacher Grabber is overkill for the situation and lacks versatile use.

Leg Lifter Strap

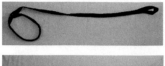
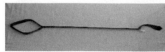

This item makes moving the operative leg easy and assists with doing exercises that involve moving it to gain flexibility and strength. Use of this item is necessary to get in and out of bed early in the recovery period. Keep this item near the bedside. Both items pictured work the same, though I prefer the non-flexible loop.

Sock Aid

I have two kinds.

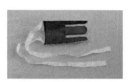

A flexible one.

Provided by the occupational therapist, is easier for me to use. I struggle with it, but not as much as with the rigid plastic one.

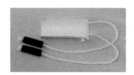

A rigid plastic one.

I can't get it to work well for me. I think the rigid plastic one may be better for people with larger feet.

Long-handled Shoehorn

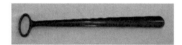

This item can also be used to peel socks off and as a scratcher. Techniques are listed later on but use for scratching is up to your itchy places.

Gel Ice Packs (or Hot and Cold Packs)

I recommend a large size pack that can be frozen or microwaved and includes a cover. Get two, so you will not need to wait for a pack to re-freeze. Be careful to avoid cutting off blood flow when using any straps to hold the ice pack cover to your body at the surgical site.

Long-handled Sponge (or Long-handled Scrub Brush)

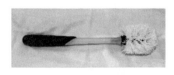

I did not use the Long-handled Sponge as I found it too bulky to get in between my toes. I improvised by cleaning my feet with a Long-handled Scrub Brush.

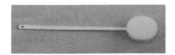

I assure you that the picture is not of a toilet brush. It is scratchy to use but it gets the job done and I was not driving anywhere to shop for something different.

Bathtub Transfer Bench

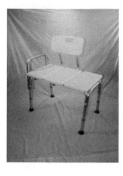

I did not use the Bathtub Transfer Bench in the bathroom much, but I do use it. My bathing habits during my recovery are detailed later. I ask the reader to consider, "safety first," when deciding whether or not to buy this item.

Safety Bars can be attached in the shower, a wall just outside of the shower, or other areas to assist with balance if you need additional handholds in the bathroom.

Do not rely on towel racks to support your weight.

Hand-held Shower Head – A comfort item to spray your lower legs and feet with at best. Not needed.

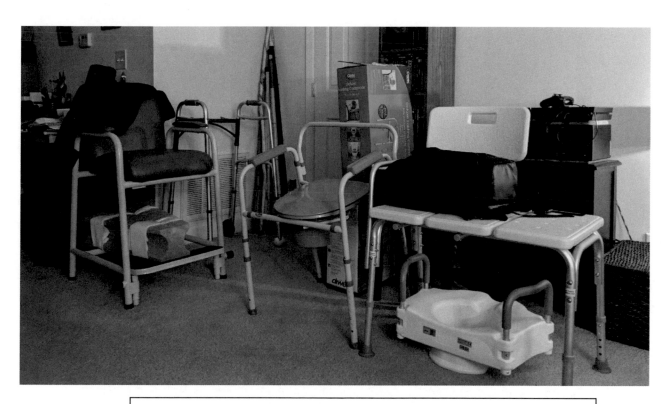

The Adaptive Equipment pile minus a few small items before I begin boxing and storing this stuff until the next surgery is needed.

Items that I recommend

Seat Riser Pillow or Hip Cushion

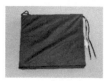
A must have to sit in a car or add to standard sized chairs to maintain Hip Precaution Guidelines. There are various thicknesses of cushion to choose from. I bought a four-inch cushion thickness and I am very happy with it. A pillow is no substitute for the consistent support this item provides with its dense foam cushion.

Pill Box – 7-day, morning and night compartments

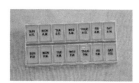
Organize morning and evening medication in advance to assist with tracking the next time for dosage. This system will streamline the primary medication regimen, but your pain medication will be taken at interval times in addition. Set timers with clocks, phones, or other devices to keep track of the schedule.

No-Rinse Wipes

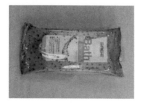
These disposable cleansing wipes are the easiest way to bathe until the shower no longer looks and feels dangerous.

Foam Wedge from the hospital

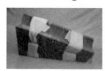
As mentioned above, the foam wedge can be used to elevate the operative leg to aid in the process of reducing swelling. I used the wedge to prevent myself from rolling over in my sleep, as well.

Walking Stick or Cane
Any walking stick or cane is useful when going for neighborhood walks and negotiating stairs while you are in recovery mode. The additional support and stability will be a welcome feeling until you regain full confidence in your movement ability.

Pre-cut Tennis Balls
Attach pre-cut tennis balls to the legs of the walker for a smoother ride.

Armchair with Seat Riser Pillow and matching height Leg Prop

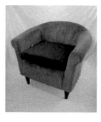 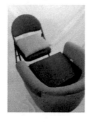

This is a combination of furniture you may already have, and it is the most comfortable way to relax outside of the bed.

Sturdy arms on the chair will assist with sitting down and standing up.

A matching height leg prop will help reduce the speed at which swelling in the lower leg will occur while sitting.

Hip Highchair

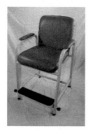

The chair is tall and made of a heavy steel frame. The chair is not comfortable to sit in for long as the chair back is too short to use as a backrest. I found this item useful as support when doing exercises because it will not topple easily, and its height allows a better posture to lean on than a folding chair. I do recommend it because of the physical therapy exercise compatibility, but I do not feel this item is necessary. I probably would not have bought it if I knew this in advance as it is pricey.

Shopping at amazon.com

Amazon.com makes finding items very easy, and home delivery is a bonus. A search for, "hip replacement," will generate a list with options to buy multiple items in the form of, "kits," and other items as "aids." Some of the kits contain more items than you need and may be more useful to patients of other medical procedures.

Adaptive Equipment Placement and Outfitting the Walker

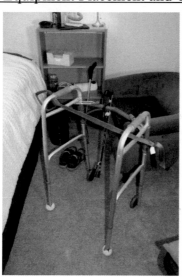

Item placement is important to making life easier during recovery.

Having as much of your frequently used items within reach is ideal.

I outfit my Walker with a Leg Lifter Strap and a Reacher Grabber Stick when I am on the go with it.

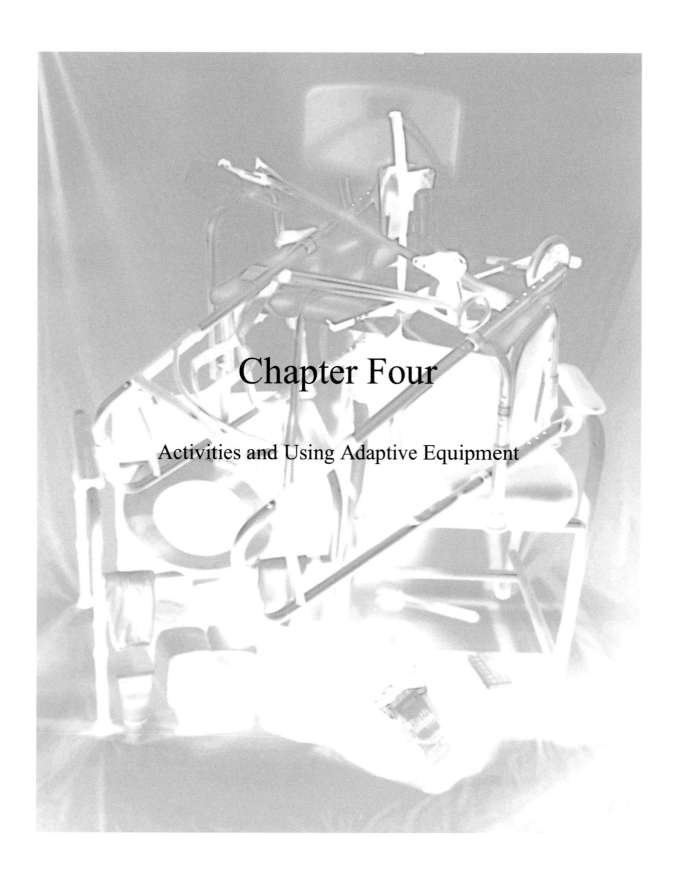

Chapter Four

Activities and Using Adaptive Equipment

Activities and Using Adaptive Equipment:

Using the Commode

There are two styles of Raised Toilet Seats pictured in the recommended Adaptive Equipment list I was given by the orthopaedic department. One seat attaches to the commode, the other sits on top of its own frame, allowing it to be used away from the bathroom. Both styles of Raised Toilet Seats have handles to assist with sitting down and getting up. The style of Raised Toilet Seat that sits on top of its own frame has the advantage of being adjustable. The seat assembly comes with a bucket to facilitate use outside of the bathroom, but its use is optional. Placing the frame over the commode with just the seat works great. In addition to adjusting to the size of the patient, the front and back legs of the frame can be set at different heights to tilt the seat forward for more comfort and flexibility to conform with the Hip Precaution Guidelines. Adjust the seat and it's frame for your comfort before you go to the hospital.

> I first bought the seat that attaches to the commode and set it up prior to surgery. The seat seemed to make sense when I tried it out. When I get home from surgery and practice using it, I discover the seat does not allow me to use correct hip precautions when sitting down. Sitting on the seat, my legs would bend at the hip near 90 degrees and my feet were not fully planted on the floor. It is a very painful posture, especially when getting up. I am 5'8'', and the commode I use is a standard size, so maybe this seat is for taller patients or shorter toilets. My wife goes out to get the other style of the Raised Toilet Seat. She finds it at Walmart. Luckily, I did not have a bowel emergency while waiting to set up the new seat. If sitting down in the bathroom is your thing get the right seat.

Use the Raised Toilet Seat – Watch on YouTube (see how in References.)

Make sure the toilet paper is within easy reach.

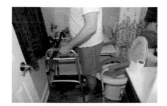 1 – Line your back up to the Raised Toilet Seat with the Walker.

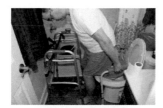 2 – Reach behind you, grasp the handles on the seat and begin slowly sitting down while supporting your weight with your arms.

> If at any time you feel extra discomfort evaluate your movement as you proceed. I will trust that you do not need me to demonstrate what to do to remove clothing and other actions involved here. A Reacher Grabber Stick may be of use, and there are instructions for undressing and dressing in another section.

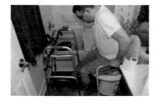 3 – Slightly extend the operative leg to help avoid using it. Be careful not to bend too much at the waist and support your body with your arms until fully seated and in position.

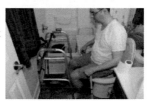 4 – Do your business after you pull down your pants and undies and pull them back up after you are done.

5 – To get up support your weight with your arms using the handles of the seat until you can grasp the walker to support you as finish standing up. Be mindful to avoid putting pressure on the operative leg.

Into the Toilet, a patient perspective fiction story.

Into the Toilet – a film noir tale of woe

The first night home after the surgery set the pace for the next two weeks. My nurse is a sweet thing, but the schedule she enforces is harsh. My mind is in a twilight state with pills every four hours, and slowly inhaling measured stale air with an Incentive Spirometer every quarter of an hour. The timetable for care is disorienting. The breath thing is my responsibility at night, so I can cheat, do, or explore because getting good sleep is a challenge. There is more freedom here than in the hospital, as intravenous tethers no longer attach me to a wall. While the nurse is away, I walk a path lit by dim nightlights to the bathroom, leaning on a rolling cage, to practice taking a dump when I know relief is days away. Gripping the handles of the attached Raised Toilet Seat, I lower my body to discover a new form of pain.

Get On and Off of a Bed – Watch on YouTube (see how in References.)

You might need to adjust your strategy for this activity if you had both of your hips replaced.

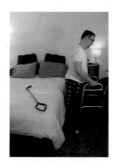 1 - Place the Leg Lifter Strap on the bed and line up your back to the bed using the Walker.

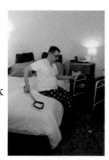 2 - Sit on the bed, move the Walker away and pick up the Leg Lifter Strap.

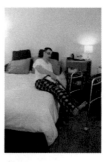 3 - Ensnare the foot of the operative leg with the Leg Lifter Strap and gently lift the leg onto the bed while leaning back a little.

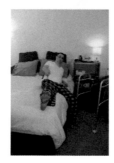 4 - Once the operative leg is on the bed position it to allow room for the other leg.

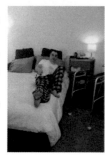 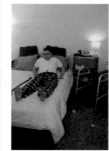 5 - Adjust for comfort using your arms and scooting your body into place.

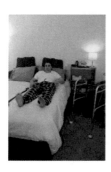

6 – To get off of the bed simply do the steps in reverse.

Select the bed you will use ahead of the surgery. Measure the height of the bed from the floor to the top of the mattress, note the side of the bed you will use in relation to the operative leg, and make a record of this information to share with an occupational therapist. Plan to place items you will use frequently close to the bed, preferably within an arm's reach.

Sit Down In and Get Up from an Armchair
The Armchair will need a Seat Riser Pillow or be of the proper height for Hip Precaution Guidelines.

Sit Down – Watch on YouTube (see how in References.)

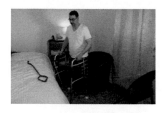

1 - Begin by standing in front of the Armchair using the Walker.

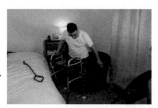

2 - Reach behind you with one hand to begin transferring your weight to the arms of the chair.

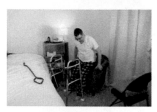

3 - Once you have both hands supporting your weight on the arms of the chair begin to gently sit down. Slightly extend the operative leg to help avoid using it.

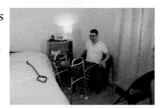

4 - It is more comfortable to also prop your leg up while seated. This will also help reduce the speed of swelling in the lower part of the leg.

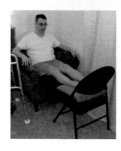

I improvise a way to prop up my leg using a folding chair and a pillow to match the height of the seat of the Armchair and keep the walker within reach for getting up. I use the Leg Lifter Strap to help position the operative leg until I feel I do not need to use it. I do not remain seated for long as the need to move and do exercises to reduce the swelling of the operative leg keeps me busy. – Watch on YouTube (see how in References.)

Get Up – Watch on YouTube (see how in References.)

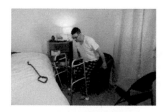

1 - Position the Walker in front of you. Place your hands on the arms of the chair and use your arms to support your weight as you stand up.

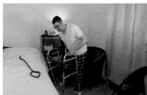

2 - Grasp the Walker with one hand and then the other as you get up. Slightly extend the operative leg to help avoid using it.

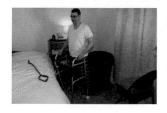

3 - Once standing it's off to the races! I like to outfit the Walker with a Leg Lifter Strap and a Reacher Grabber. The chance I will need one or the other when I get to where I go is high.

I feel it necessary to mention I do not use the Walker for long. While it is necessary to provide the reader with an accurate account of my recovery experience, I stress that all of it is temporary. Each day the confidence to move on my own grows and when the swelling is under control, I am as comfortable as I can be.

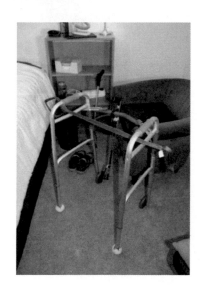

Get Dressed and Undressed

Getting dressed and undressed requires a Reacher Grabber Stick, Sock Aid, and a Long-handled Shoehorn. Shoes need to have loosely pre-tied laces or Elastic Shoelaces for best performance and safety. Place all clothing items you need within easy reach and use the Reacher Grabber Stick to retrieve and move the items. Sit on the edge of a chair that is the correct height to follow the Hip Precaution list.

Put Socks On – Watch on YouTube (see how in References.)

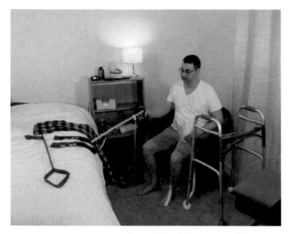

1 - With the Sock Aid in hand retrieve a sock with the Reacher Grabber Stick.

The socks I use for the photos and video are two toned in color and the bottom of the socks are black. Please note the orientation of the black portion of the sock to gain a perspective of how I turn the sock to complete the task.

Propping the Sock Aid against your stomach is the best way to make the task of putting the sock onto it easy.

Chuckle all you want pervs.

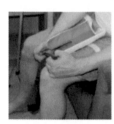

2 – Begin pulling the sock onto the Sock Aid with the top of the sock on the open side of the Sock Aid.

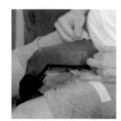

3 – As you continue to pull the sock onto the Sock Aid avoid overlapping the folds of the sock as the overlaps will prevent a smooth slide off of the Sock Aid later.

4 – Thread the sock onto the Sock Aid and leave some room at the toe.

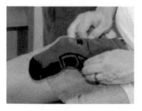
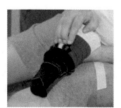
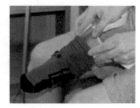

5 – When the sock is fully on the Sock Aid smooth out any overlapping folds and widen the open end to prepare for putting the sock on your foot.

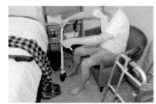

6 – Move the Sock Aid into position and begin pulling the sock on.

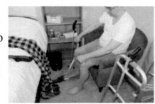

7 – Getting the sock on as you pull the handle straps of the Sock Aid will likely require on the fly adjustments and using a Reacher Grabber Stick to grasp and adjust the sock as you go.

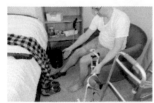

8 – The sock might not cooperate and come off of the Sock Aid before the process is complete.

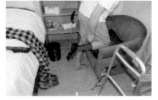

9 – To fix the sock stand up, turn around, kneel the sock problem leg on the Hip Precaution height chair seat and reach around to pull the sock the rest of the way on.

Take Socks Off – Watch on YouTube (see how in References.)

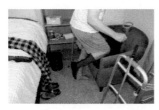 1 – Kneel on a Hip Precaution height chair seat and have the Long-handled Shoehorn ready to use.

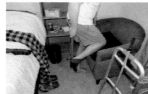 2 – Reach around to pull the sock down then finish removing the sock by sliding the Long-handled Shoehorn into the sock to push the sock off.

Put Pants On (or undies) – Watch on YouTube (see how in References.)

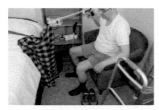 1 – Retrieve the pants with a Reacher Grabber Stick and position them on the floor in front of you with the waist of the pants front side up.

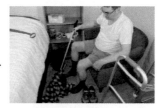 2 – Use the Reacher Grabber Stick to help start putting the pant leg of the operative leg on.

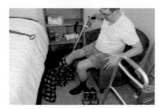 3 – Do not lean down to pull up the pants. Use the Reacher Grabber Stick to get the pants within easy reach.

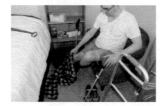 4 – When you can reach the pants without leaning over hold the pants in place to put the non-operative leg into its pant leg.

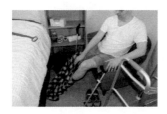 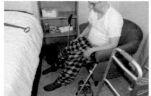 5 – Pull the pants up as far as comfortable and free your feet from the bottoms of the pants legs. Stand up to finish pulling the pants up.

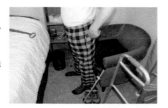

Take Pants Off (or undies) – Watch on YouTube (see how in References.)

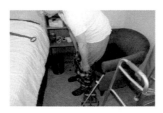 1 – In a standing position push the pants down as far as you can while bending as little as possible.

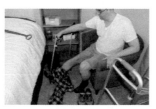 2 – Sit down and finish removing the pants with the Reacher Grabber Stick. Free the non-operative leg first and then the pants from the operative leg.

Put Shoes On – Watch on YouTube (see how in References.)

Bend at the waist as little as possible.

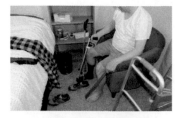 1 – Place the shoes close to where you will sit to put them on and have the Reacher Grabber Stick and Long-handled Shoehorn ready to use.

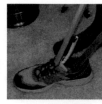 2 – Grab the shoe's tongue with the Reacher Grabber Stick and place the end of the Long-handled Shoehorn inside the shoe at the heel.

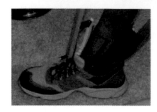 3 – Insert your foot keeping a grip on the shoe's tongue with the Reacher Grabber Stick. Pin the shoe to the floor with the Long-handled Shoehorn as you slide the heel of your foot down it into the shoe.

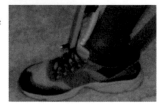 4 – Finish sliding your foot into the shoe.

Take Shoes Off – Watch on YouTube (see how in References.)

I recommend using this technique with both shoes to avoid bending at the waist.

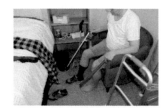 1 – Sit down with a Reacher Grabber Stick and a Long-handled Shoehorn in hand.

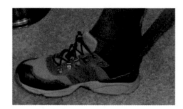 2 – Insert the Long-handled Shoehorn into the shoe at the heel and push the shoe off.

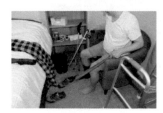 3 – Use the Reacher Grabber Stick to move the shoes and any other items out of the way before you stand up.

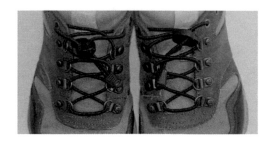 Elastic Shoelaces make the tasks of putting shoes on and taking them off a breeze. Regular shoelaces can be loosely pre-tied. Adjust your shoelace solution before surgery.

Tying shoelaces while wearing the shoes is not an option during your recovery from surgery.

Bathing

Protect the Surgical Site

Following surgery, the surgical site is protected with an adhesive bandage you need to keep dry. I follow the instructions I am given by my doctors concerning this topic to the letter and beyond. The surgical site requires a new covering every day until the staples are removed. My wife helps to measure the incision site and buys two sizes of bandages at a CVS store. A large rectangular bandage to cover the long incision scar and a smaller rectangular bandage to cover an adjacent incision area.

Twelve days after surgery, I go to my general practitioner doctor to have the staples removed from the surgical site. After the staples are gone, the doctor covers the mostly healed incision scar with Steri-Strips. The incision scar is very scabby, and the Steri-Strips will fall off as the skin they are attached to flakes off. The doctor recommends I do not get the Steri-Strips wet and in general to keep the whole incision scar area dry until the Steri-Strips fall off.

I decide to protect my Steri-Strips from rubbing off early by taping gauze over them, changing the gauze and first aid tape every other day. Seeing the progress of the scabs and scar as they become less angry looking reassures me that waiting to wash the area is wise. I do not want to peel off a scab and extend the healing time by mistake or make a part of the scar worse by picking at it.

Most of my Steri-Strips fell off within 14 days. Over time lint will adhere to the tape glue and become a nuisance. You can remove the lint and glue with rubbing alcohol, cotton balls, and your fingernails. Wet a cotton ball with rubbing alcohol and rub the glue until it begins to give. Keep rubbing to remove or scrape it off with a fingernail, just be careful when getting close to any Steri-Strips that are still attached to you.

A do it yourself technique to apply a gauze bandage:

Cut double the length of gauze needed, then fold it in half.

Make strips of first aid tape and attach them to the gauze keeping the exposed ends glue side up.

Leave a half inch of gauze loose at the ends to prevent it pulling free from the tape later.

Carefully press the gauze with tape into position over the Steri-Strips, and smooth tape ends against your skin. Use a mirror to check your work.

Avoid attaching the first aid tape to the Steri-Strips.

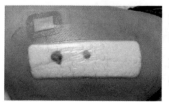

Bandages covering a long incision scar and a smaller adjacent area.

Leakage is normal but go to the doctor if the amount is worrisome.

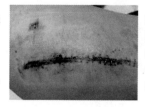

Staples or stitches? My surgeon chose staples. Other surgeons may use stitches.

Sorry, there are no pictures of the Steri-Strips and gauze bandage. I did not know I would be making this book at the time.

My personal hygiene routine

I do not take a standing shower until 26 days after surgery. On that day, when I peel off the gauze taped over the incision scar, the last of the Steri-Strips are flaking off the scar, so I begin removing the tape glue and lint stuck to my skin. The lint packed glue takes some work to rub and scrape off with isopropyl alcohol, cotton balls, and my fingernails. When I finish the job, I realize with glee that I am now waterproof! It is the best shower in my personal history of showering.

Before that happy day, I start my hygiene routine by standing in front of the bathroom sink with the Walker in easy reach. Shaving my face and brushing my teeth are no-brainers. To wash my hair, I run the water in the sink to the right temperature and lean over the sink, with care to not bend too much at the waist, and scoop water onto my head with my hands. Then I lather my hair with shampoo, scooping water to rinse until I am satisfied. This process is messy with splashing, and I switched to using the kitchen sink because of its larger basin to catch water and taller counter height. I did not always remember to make sure a towel is in reach and often made a wet trail while retrieving it.

Washing my body is a more involved process, with my feet being the biggest challenge. When I get home from the hospital, I decide to be unwashed for as long as I can tolerate, and I like being clean. I learn about No-Rinse Wipes during a phone call to a family member and have my wife go get some. I use the No-Rinse Wipes while sitting on my Bathtub Transfer Bench, which is in my living room because the bathroom is very small in our apartment. There is nobody at home to shock with my nakedness. The No-Rinse Wipes are easy to use to wash what I can reach of my body, but they leave a residue on my skin that annoys me, so I use a damp washcloth to rinse.

Cleaning my body gets easier as its healing progresses, and I rely less on the Walker to get around. I place the Bathtub Transfer Bench in the shower tub when I need to wash my feet and return it to the living room after, so it is not in the way of using the Raised Toilet Seat at the commode. While sitting on the Bathtub Transfer Bench in the tub, I dip my feet in a bucket of soapy water and wash them with a Long-Handled Scrubber, as the Long-Handled Sponge can't get in between my toes. I rinse my feet under the bathtub faucet being careful not to bend too much at the waist while turning the water on, adjusting it for temperature, and turning the water off.

If you must use the shower

Personal hygiene is going to take some planning and the use of a few Adaptive Equipment items for the first six weeks after surgery. Necessary Adaptive Equipment items include Walker, Bathtub Transfer Bench, and a Long-handled Sponge (or Long-handled Scrub Brush). Safety Bars can be installed for additional support to prevent falling. Do not use towel racks or other bath fixtures for balancing. Safety is a priority, and additionally, the surgical site and bandage must remain dry while bathing.

> Tasks that take place in front of a sink are easy to do because you can lean on the sink for support, your hygiene items are easy to reach, and water is controllable. Washing your hair and body will require more preparation and care. A Hand-held Shower Head is useful for controlling water while you are in the bathtub, but I am not inspired to buy one.
>
> I buy a Bathtub Transfer Bench to use because it provides more safety and comfort while getting in and out of a bathtub than a Bathtub Chair.

Use the Bathtub Transfer Bench – Watch on YouTube (see how in References.)

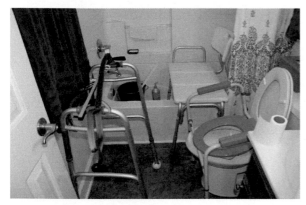

1 – Place all of the items you will need in and around the tub before you attempt to bathe using the Bathtub Transfer Bench.

In the tub I have a bucket, Long-handle Scrub Brush (and Sponge), wash cloth, and soap/ bodywash.

The towel is in easy reach on a towel rack, and there is no bath mat to be a floor hazard.

The Walker holds a Reacher Grabber Stick and a Leg Lifter Strap.

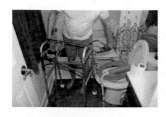

2 – After you are in position with the Walker begin to sit down on the end of the Bathtub Transfer Bench. I am using the Walker and a handle on the Raised Toilet Seat to steady myself.

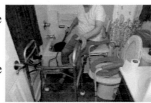

3 – Once seated retrieve the Leg Lifter Strap and move the Walker out of the way.

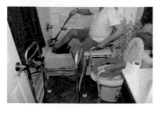

4 – Snag the foot of the operative leg with the Leg Lifter Strap and gently assist the leg into the tub. I lean back slightly while doing this and use a handle on the Raised Toilet Seat for support.

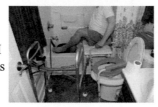

5 – Place the Leg Lifter Strap in easy reach, slide across the seat using your arms, and move the good leg into the tub.

Cover the surgical site bandage with plastic wrap and seal the wrap with tape if you anticipate excessive splashing. Do not be a daredevil and attempt a standing shower. A slip and a fall are activities you want to prevent. The precariousness of the bathtub experience will make an impression with your instinct for self-preservation.

Get Out of the Tub – Watch on YouTube (see how in References.)

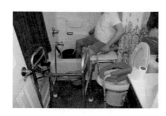

1 – Move the good leg out of the tub and use your arms to slide over the seat and retrieve the Leg Lifter Strap.

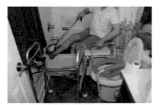

2 – Free the operative leg from the tub using the Leg Lifter Strap. When both feet are on the floor pull the Walker closer and use it to stand up.

> To avoid bending too much at the waist while bathing I fill the bucket with warm soapy water before I get in to wash my feet. I use a Long-handled Scrub Brush as the Sponge does not get in between my toes. Reaching to turn the water on and off while sitting on the Shower Transfer Bench is uncomfortable. I am eager to get out of the tub after my feet are rinsed.

The Pond, a patient perspective fiction story.

<u>The Pond</u> – a fantasy tale from the bathroom forest

My body feels long and brittle as if I were a human and tree hybrid creature. My feet are itchy roots that branches cannot unearth to scratch. My trunk can sway, but not bend, as I sit on a Shower Transfer Bench in a tiny slick walled dry pond. I uproot a wooden leg with a Leg Lifter Strap, gently guiding it over the tall shore, and lower it into the pond. Sliding into position on the bench, I move the other more flesh feeling leg into the pond easily. I need to wash the dirt off of my roots, but I can't get my trunk wet, and I dare not fall.

Water in the walled dry pond can be conjured in two ways. Sky water is not safe for the trunk, so I opt for wall water. I conjure wall water to fill a hollow beside me to make lather. I scrub my roots holding a bristle-like branch that extends my reach, dipping it into the lather hollow beforehand. Once my roots are lathered, I conjure the wall water to rinse them off in a stream. I am now a human and tree hybrid creature stuck on a bench in a wet tiny slick walled pond. There is no conjuring an exit.

I slide across the bench and free the leg of flesh. The Leg Lifter Strap is where I left it, propped against the tall shore of the pond. Snagging the roots of the wooden leg with the Leg Lifter Strap, I free it from the pond and prepare to restore my height. I grasp a handle on the bench with a branch and use my flesh leg to lift my trunk and wooden leg while I reach out with another branch to grasp a Walker to gain stability as I rise.

As I leave this perilous environment, the bark falls away from the wooden parts of my body as my head reaches its canopy, my roots become feet, and I am no longer in danger of slipping, falling, or sabotaging the surgical bandage on my hip. I will return to this pond only when my feet disgust me enough to risk my safety again. I do still bathe sitting on the Shower Transfer Bench as I recover from my surgery, using No-Rinse Wipes, but not in the pond.

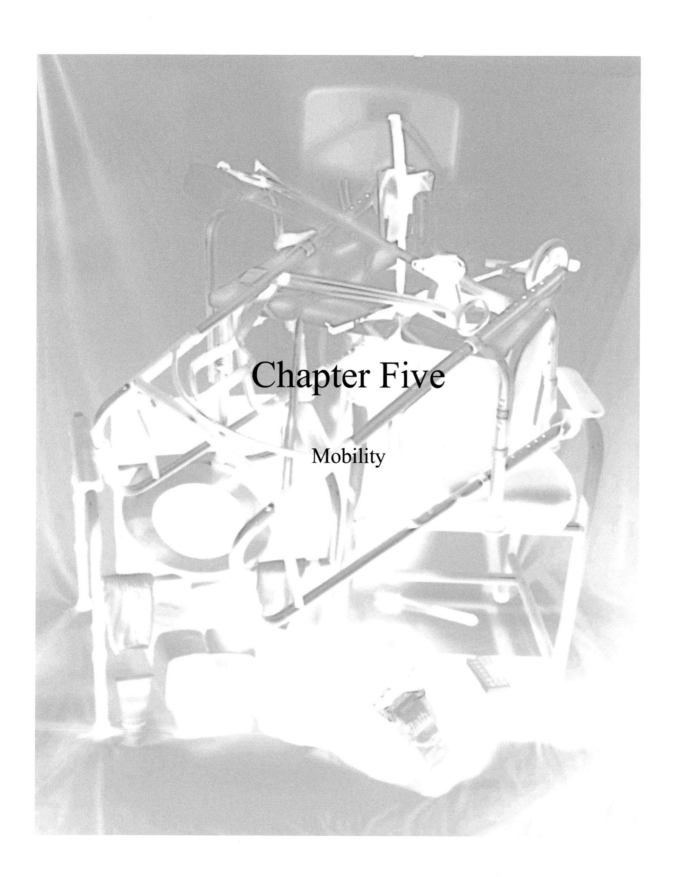

Chapter Five

Mobility

Mobility

Get Out of the Hospital

The ability to get around on your feet after surgery will advance in stages. A physical therapist will guide you and make sure you can get in and out of the hospital bed safely. The need to pee will be like clockwork at least every half hour once you are hooked up to a drip IV. Dehydration is a side effect of the surgery, and you will want to drink lots of water on impulse, too. A nurse must be called to observe that you can safely get up and get back into bed, but privacy is respected while you do the deed.

> It is at this stage of my hospital stay when my care experience is a little dicey because of the length of time since my last meal. Remember to have someone with you that can go out and bring you something to eat. If the hospital is no longer serving food, it is OK for someone to leave the hospital and bring food back for you.
>
> You will want to have water, snacks, candy, and the Chapstick within easy reach when you are lying on the hospital bed. My lips are very dry and cracked after surgery due to the use of an oxygen tube. While it is thoughtful that the Patient Program Class swag bag contains Chapstick, I wisely bring a fancy medicated moisturizing lip balm.
>
> Bring a book, electronic devise, or something low maintenance to use for entertainment and keep it close to the bed. Headphones or earbuds are good accessories to have. A television is in the room, but you might have room mates. A nurse with medication will interrupt your entertainment or rest every four hours overnight to check on your pain needs and condition.

A physical therapist will stop in shortly after you have breakfast the morning after your surgery and instruct you to perform mobility tasks. Completing the tasks to the satisfaction of the physical therapist is the first checkbox on a list of prerequisites to qualify for release from the hospital.

Using a Walker to go down a hallway and back is the first task. The physical therapist observes how steady you are and that you are not turning your operative leg inward at the foot while you walk. The therapist gives tips on how to be mindful of keeping the operative leg in a proper posture during your recovery.

Going up and down a set of mock stairs with guard rails is the next task. To climb the staircase, I learn to step first with my good leg and bring the operative leg to the same step after. I go up the stairs step by step, turn around on the top platform and descend stepping with the operative leg first and then the good leg, step by step until I am on the floor. The guard rails of the stairs get a lot of use when taking the steps. Walking feels really awkward the day after surgery.

Climbing into and out of a mock car is the last task. The process involves lining up your backside with an open car door, sitting down on the car seat, and pivoting one leg into the car at a time. To correct positioning while seated, you use your arms to lift and scoot your body into place. Once you are out of the mock car, the physical therapist escorts you back to the hospital room.

A visit from an occupational therapist is next. The occupational therapist will guide you through another list of tasks, some of which require the use of Adaptive Equipment. The list of tasks include: get off and on a bed using a Leg Lifter Strap, use a Reacher Grabber Stick to put on pants, use a Reacher Grabber Stick and a Long-handled Shoehorn to put on and take off socks and shoes, and demonstrate you can sit on and get up from the hospital room's bathroom toilet – it has side handles and is the correct height for hip precaution guidelines. These are the last tests to pass before you are cleared for discharge from the hospital.

The occupational therapist provides the Adaptive Equipment for you to perform the list of tasks. It is still unclear to me if patients can expect to keep the items or if the items are only for use in the hospital. I take some of the items even though I already have similar items at home because I like them more, and I did not buy a Long-handled Sponge. Perhaps the medical program you attend will be less vague about what items it will provide to patients.

Mobility at Home

Walking is an essential activity during recovery. You use a Walker to get around for a surprisingly short time. Just be smart about when you need extra support. It is a process to gain confidence while moving. A Cane or Walking Stick is an excellent companion to bring when walking outdoors as negotiating stairs will feel dicey without extra support, especially if there are no handrails. Pay attention to your body as it heals, and you will recognize when to stop using the Adaptive Equipment.

Pain medication is the last obstacle to vehicular mobility. The legal process for driving a vehicle under the influence is not an activity you want to add to the final stages of recovery. "Cabin fever is a bother, the world outside is so inviting, and some places take too long to walk to," you may say. The world can wait until the doctor clears you to drive six weeks after surgery.

Protecting the hip implant from wear and tear dictates the activities you can do from now on. The surgeon will warn you of a list of activities that will accelerate the need to replace the hip implant. A short list of restricted activities includes running, jumping, and lifting more than forty pounds. A short list of permitted activities includes light hiking, biking, swimming, and golf. Exercise is encouraged as weight gain will also shorten the life span of the hip implant. Going to a gym that has instructors familiar with patient recovery is a wise choice. The hip implant will last more than fifteen years if you behave well.

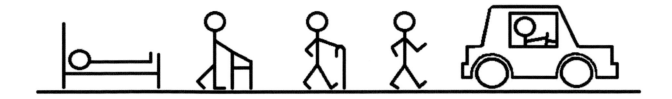

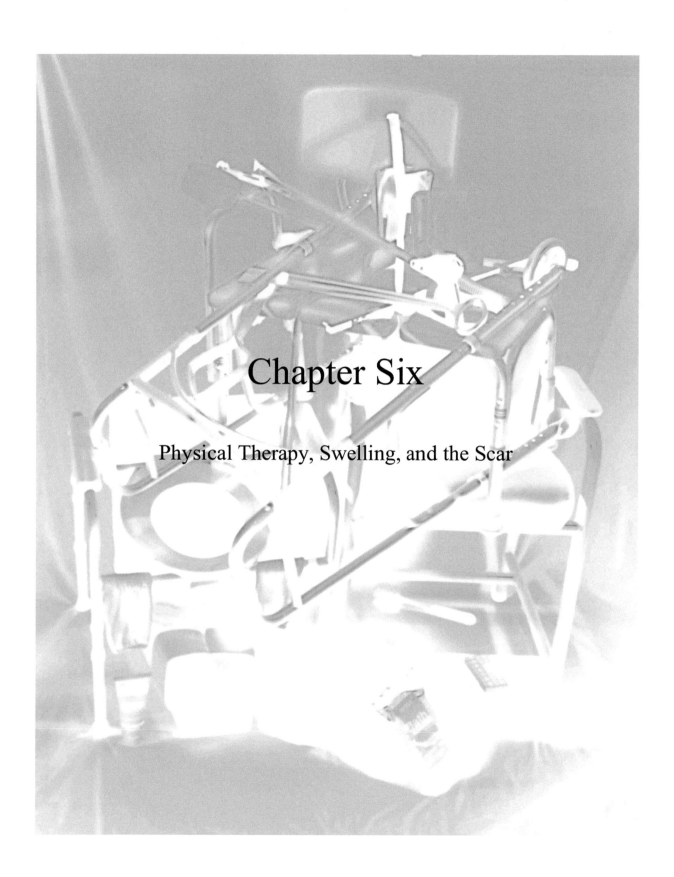

Chapter Six

Physical Therapy, Swelling, and the Scar

Physical Therapy, Swelling, and the Scar

Physical Therapy is not as intense as the name implies, but it is a daily home activity enhanced by professional therapy sessions twice a week. The exercises are not complicated but do present a challenge because they target the areas affected by surgery that need regrowth and strengthening. The hardest aspect of physical therapy may be that it needs to be a daily routine. The home exercise list takes a little more than half an hour to complete. Weather permitting, I like to walk outside for at least fifteen minutes before I begin the routine. The order you do the exercises can affect your stamina to complete specific tasks or aid in reducing swelling.

The list of exercises recommended will change with your healing progression. A nurse provides me with a list of exercises and some instructions before I leave the hospital. Understanding how these initial exercises reduce swelling is crucial.

The exercises that I learn to do at the physical therapy center are not always things I can do at home. The physical therapist will provide you with exercises you can do at home and update the activities as you improve. The exercises require proper form and technique to be effective. A physical therapist is a valuable source of knowledge and will ensure you are not wasting effort.

Swelling is an issue at some point after surgery. I experience sudden significant swelling several days after surgery. I get instructions from my physical therapist as soon as I can. I am not doing several things correctly or enough. I need to apply icepacks to the surgery site, not the location of the swelling. The swelling I have is below the knee and requires doing specific exercises more frequently and elevating the operative leg correctly to provide relief. It takes a couple of days for me to get the swelling under control after I learn the right things to do.

> Sitting in a chair for too long is an issue. Resting the operative leg on an equal height leg prop slows the rate of swelling. Getting up and moving around every fifteen minutes or when stiffness starts to occur helps. Doing the lying down exercises are the most effective activity for swelling reduction, though. Performing a consistent routine is an evolving process, but once the swelling is relieved, it is easy to maintain control. Swelling is a temporary side effect of surgery and healing will solve all of it soon.

Swelling is reduced by performing exercises in a specific order. Doing seated or standing exercises first and the ones lying down last worked best. The exercises lying down are the ones that help drain fluid from the leg and should be done as often as possible to manage and reduce swelling. Lying down exercises, such as ankle pumps, can enhance their benefit by elevating the operative leg while doing them. The Foam Wedge I bring home from the hospital is useful to elevate the operative leg. The physical therapist recommends I use a steeper angle to elevate the leg which I achieve at home using the Leg Lifter Strap to support the operative leg while lying down and rotating the position of the Foam Wedge.

Use the Foam Wedge – sorry, no video. Finding the right angle involves a lot of improvisation.

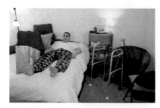

1 – Get into a comfortable lying down position on a bed with the Foam Wedge next to your operative leg and have the Leg Lifter Strap in hand. The floor is a bad option due to the careful positioning you need to adhere to during the early stages of healing. Getting up off of the floor is a surprisingly difficult thing to do.

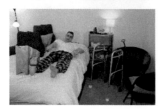

2 – Snag the foot of the operative leg with the Leg Lifter Strap and gently begin to lift the leg to the height of the Foam Wedge.

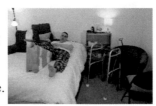

3 – Push the Foam Wedge under the operative leg and rest the leg on the wedge. Start with ankle pump exercises to reduce swelling.

> The physical therapist recommends I use a steeper angle for elevating the leg which I achieve at home using the Leg Lifter Strap to support the operative leg while lying down and rotating the position of the Foam Wedge.

Care for the scar is also a part of the physical therapy I learn towards the end of my sessions. The physical therapist uses massage lotion and a rubbing technique that pushes the skin on either side of the scar towards the seam of the scar itself. The sensation is a little strange and the scar pops like you are pushing out air bubbles. The goal is to hydrate the scar tissue to keep it pliable and soft to reduce the profile of the scar as it heals. I buy the same lotion the physical therapist uses in as small a quantity as I can at amazon.com.

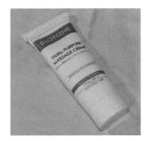

> I am not fond of gyms. I choose to walk a lot, continue the exercises I learn at the physical therapy gym I attend during recovery, and I buy a set of resistance loops and bands for low impact resistance training. I contact my orthopaedics department to make sure any new exercises I intend to do will not impact the hip implant negatively.

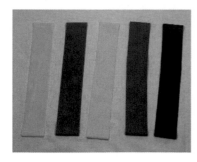

Resistance loops have different resistant strength levels and are color coded. My set includes a storage bag.

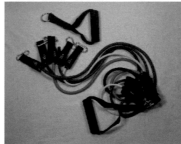

Resistance bands also have color code for resistance levels and allow a large range of exercise possibilities. You can buy bands separately. I buy a set with a storage bag.

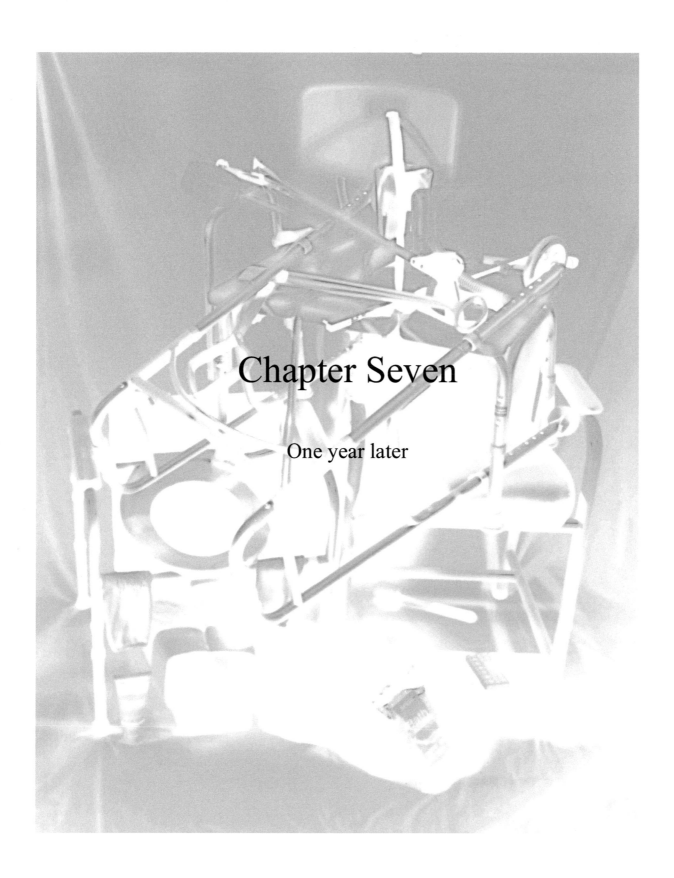

Chapter Seven

One year later

One year later

I am still adjusting to living with a hip implant a year after my hip replacement surgery. The hardest part is remembering to not push the limits of the forty-pound lifting and pulling restriction. It is so easy to do a task without thinking because I feel like my old self again. I am thankful my workmates help me by moving things I can't or shouldn't. Standing for any length of time is not painful, and I no longer need to think about each step I take. I love my Elastic Shoe Laces, and all of my shoes and boots now have them except my work shoes that wear out more frequently.

I discover other aspects of life need a tweak, too. I am aware dentist visits require antibiotics, but the effects of which require me to take two days off – the day of the appointment and the day after to allow diarrhea to run its course. Sorry for, "too much information," my dentist insists not all folks are affected the same way. Airport security is not an issue. Signs are posted reminding you to let the security screeners know you have a metal implant. I make foam riser cushions to elevate my living room furniture, so my seating options are not too low for comfort. I am sure there will be new scenarios to adapt to over time, as well.

I gain some weight from being less active while adjusting to physical restrictions, the weather, and my own faults. I refuse to buy new pants. I need to be more vigilant to walk and exercise outside of my work. I will not pay for a gym membership. I buy two kinds of resistance bands and make exercise routine guide books using the resources the bands come with and supplement them with YouTube videos. All exercises are low impact, and some are the same exercises the physical therapy place teaches during recovery. I contact my orthopaedic doctor to make sure the exercises I have in mind to do will not damage the hip implant assembly. Surprisingly, jump rope is OK in addition to jogging in place. I do not intend to do jump rope. I just test the subject with the doctor.

I find solutions to use my kayaks that do not involve buying a different vehicle, but I need to replace the car top racks I have. Some products provide a lift-assist method to get the kayaks up and secure on top of a vehicle. I choose the economical Malone J-Loader™ J-style kayak carriers paired with a Malone Telos-XL™ kayak lift-assist set. A fancier option is the Thule Hullavator Pro™ which is spring loaded to provide automatic lift-assist. I transport two kayaks, and the Hullavator rack is potentially too wide to fit two sets on the roof racks of a vehicle. Both styles of kayak lift-assist products require the user to lift a kayak to the middle height of the vehicle to load them on the racks. My solution is to buy a folding metal luggage rack to use as a fulcrum, and I use a kayak cart to move the boat around. After getting things lined up and spaced along the side of the vehicle, I lift one end of the kayak and rest it on the luggage rack. Then I lift the other end and pivot it into the kayak rack. The end of the kayak on the luggage rack will easily pivot into the rack on its end. Each kayak lift-assist product has instructions on how to finish the job of putting the kayak on top of the car from there.

Changing my career is a work in progress. I am OK with what I do in the restaurant for now, but I need to find a way to move on. With luck, this writing project will be the start of my new profession. I am working on some fiction stories with a mysterious sci-fi flair. My other hip needs the same surgery. I will wait until it starts to bother me, but not as long a time as the first hip. I definitely want to be in better physical shape before the next surgery to avoid additional weight gain and speed recovery by toning the necessary muscle groups ahead of time.

I hope my story and this book soothes any anxiety or mystery you may have concerning the need for hip replacement surgery and provides you with ideas for your strategy to prepare, recover, and adjust to life after your hip replacement surgery. Your experience may require you to discover ways to continue enjoying some activities. I wish the best for you, and I know at the very least, walking without pain is something you will love to do again.

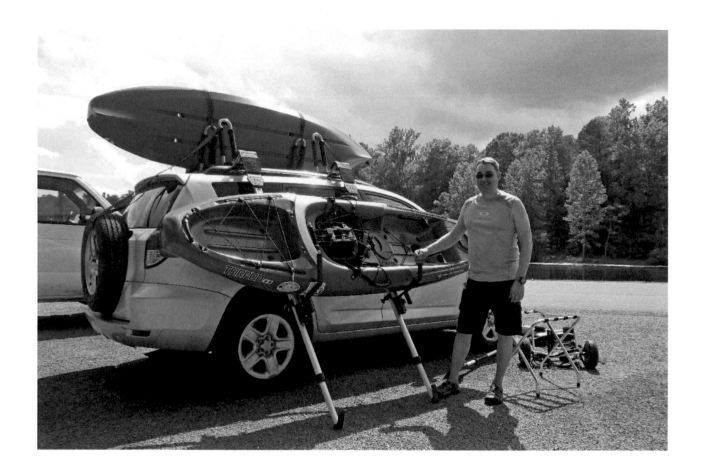

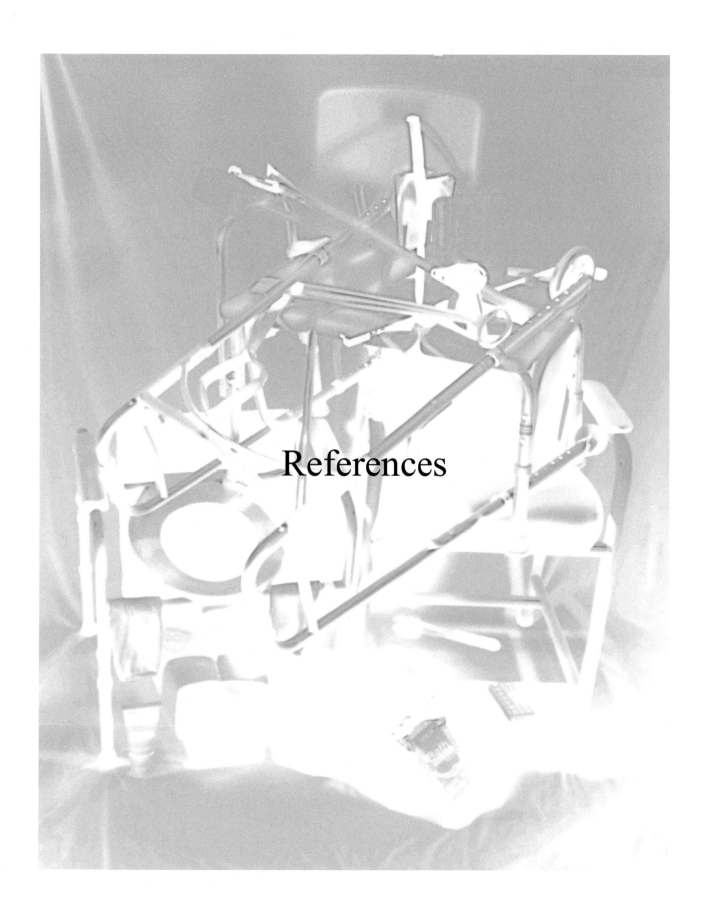

References

References

Operating Room Video

The author does not claim any rights to the operating room video. The video has a YouTube Creative Commons Attribution license (reuse allowed).

"Minimally invasive anterior hip arthroplasty, the Röttinger approach - Dr. O. Bringer."

https://www.youtube.com/watch?v=5UdtKdAejbE&list=WL&index=8&t=103s

YouTube

Search for "uduforu" at YouTube.com.

The author created videos featured in the e-book are in the "Hip Adaptive Equipment" playlist.

YouTube video website addresses:

Use the Raised Toilet Seat - https://youtu.be/RohS8E4-Dqs

Get On and Off of a Bed - https://youtu.be/FgGFJVITny4

Sit in an Armchair - https://youtu.be/cZYJyg9CH5Y

Use a Leg Prop - https://youtu.be/-qohBCtWD7w

Get Up from an Armchair - https://youtu.be/6C45ePlHx68

Put Socks On - https://youtu.be/OUJx9O5KmQw

Take Socks Off - https://youtu.be/PyVjXe2KTLE

Put Pants On (or undies) - https://youtu.be/lzS8Mg4vo2Y

Take Pants Off (or undies) - https://youtu.be/kvblW1OpvUA

Put Shoes On - https://youtu.be/ylCTMC9Vt_0

Take Shoes Off - https://youtu.be/9IsbxNwIPJw

Use the Bathtub Transfer Bench - https://youtu.be/lNw8Cj05344

Get Out of the Tub - https://youtu.be/Zxq-wIBOgks

If you have not started a medical program, I suggest the following resources for information:

American Academy of Orthopaedic Surgeons

https://orthoinfo.aaos.org

What is a total hip replacement?

https://orthoinfo.aaos.org/en/treatment/total-hip-replacement/

What to ask doctors?

https://orthoinfo.aaos.org/en/treatment/total-joint-replacement-questions-patients-should-ask-their-surgeon/

How to prepare for treatment?

https://orthoinfo.aaos.org/en/treatment/preparing-for-joint-replacement-surgery/

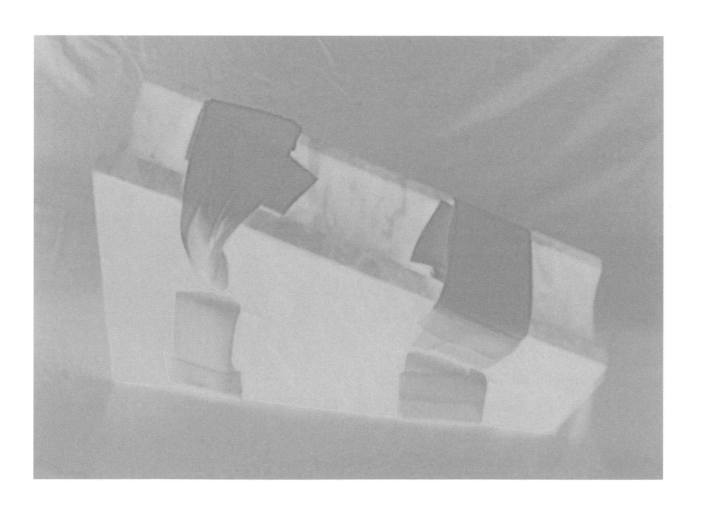

About the author

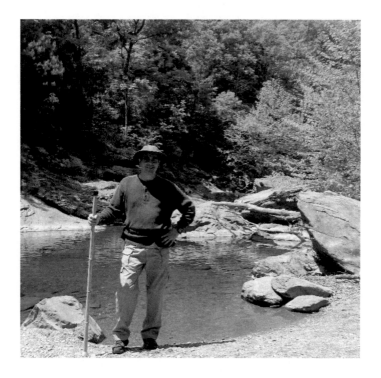

Martin E. Dodge lives in Charlottesville, Virginia with his beautiful wife, Spring.

uduforu.com

uduforu press

Visit the website to see what I'm up to.

Made in the USA
Middletown, DE
04 March 2020

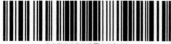

85755973R10040